Yoga Hacks

33 Essential Yoga Tips to Recharge, Refresh and Improve Your Yoga Practice—TODAY!

Olivia Summers

Published in The USA by:

Success Life Publishing

125 Thomas Burke Dr.

Hillsborough, NC 27278

ISBN-10: 1512242934

Disclaimer

Every effort has been made to accurately represent this book and its potential. Results vary with every individual, and your results may or may not be different from those depicted. No promises, guarantees or warranties, whether stated or implied, have been made that you will produce any specific result from this book. Your efforts are individual and unique, and may vary from those shown. Your success depends on your efforts, background and motivation.

The material in this publication is provided for educational and informational purposes only and is not intended as medical advice. The information contained in this book should not be used to diagnose or treat any illness, metabolic disorder, disease or health problem. Always consult your physician or health care provider before beginning any nutrition or exercise program. Use of the programs, advice, and information contained in this book is at the sole choice and risk of the reader.

Table of Contents

Introduction

Hi! My name is Olivia Summers and thank you so much for taking the time to read my book "Yoga Hacks."

First, let's start by defining the term 'hack.' What does it mean? Well, simply put it's just a modern day term used to describe a simply solution to a tricky problem. For instance, in this case the problem is not being challenged enough by your yoga practice or getting bored with your current yoga routine. The solution—or hack—in this case is the easy-to-follow tips and solutions offered up in my book.

Inside you'll find over 30 different "hacks" to help revitalize and switch up your yoga practice. If you're like me and have been practicing for awhile, things can start to feel stale. Just like anything—in the beginning things feel fun and exciting and even somewhat addicting. But after a year or more of the same old thing you can start to lose your focus and slowly you begin to wonder why you started practicing in the first place.

First of all, don't worry: the feelings you have are completely normal and I want to reassure you that there *is* something you can do about it. Just like a fizzled out love connection, your feelings toward your yoga practice can be rekindled. All it takes is a little newness and excitement to be reintroduced to help you get back on your game and fall in love with yoga all over again.

This book is your answer to sparking a new love for yoga with simple tweaks and changes that you can implement right away.

Without a doubt, the information that you're about to read will not only improve your yoga practice, but all other aspects of your life as well—and that's what it's all about: the journey.

Hack 1: Experiment With Inversions

First though…what are they? Well, inversions are merely asanas (or poses) where your head is positioned below your heart. If you're like most yoga students and you haven't yet tried inversions, then I understand the hesitation. In class when I suggest these types of poses to my students I am often met with hesitation and a look of anxiety— sometimes even a very verbal, "Hell no."

And I get it: the idea of completely turning yourself upside down goes against our entire sense of human nature. But that doesn't necessarily mean it's a bad thing. In fact, practicing inversions on a regular basis is incredibly good for your health. Don't believe me?

Here are some benefits you can expect from getting upside down:

- Improved core strength
- Increased stamina and endurance
- Sense of accomplishment
- FUN—it makes you feel like a kid again
- Higher levels of self-confidence
- Better balance
- Elevated energy levels
- Reversed blood flow to aid in improved circulation

- Keeps your lymph moving along
- Gives you a whole new outlook on life—literally

Yes, all of these benefits and more can be experienced simply from getting upside down for a few minutes a day. Pretty impressive, right? Not to mention, the more you practice the less intimidating it becomes and the more fun you have.

So maybe now I've convinced you to give inversions a try, but you're curious about how to start.

Here are some inversion poses for you to try right away:

- Legs-Up-The-Wall Pose
- Plow Pose
- Shoulderstand
- L Stand
- Headstand
- Handstand
- Forearm Balance
- Scorpion

  The list goes on, but I think you get the idea…

Please keep in mind, however, that there are some important health factors to consider before giving inversions a try. If you have any of the following, please consult your physician before attempting any of these poses: heart conditions, high blood pressure, glaucoma, eye injuries, neck injuries, epilepsy or stroke.

Please also note that it is NOT advised to do inversions while menstruating, as these types of poses reverse the flow of blood back into our body and are believed to cause stagnant energy. This is definitely not scientifically proven by any means, but it does make sense to me to avoid doing strenuous activity during your menstrual cycle that could cause disruption in your body's cleansing process. So above all, just listen to your body and treat it with the respect that it deserves and you should be just fine.

Hack 2: Try a Fast

Fasting, much like yoga, has been around for centuries and is based in religious and spiritual practice. But also like yoga, you definitely don't have to be religious or even spiritual to give fasting a try.

You might be thinking to yourself, "Why would anyone go without food—ever?" And I used to wonder the same thing. However, after a lot of research on the subject and even several fasts under my belt at this stage in life, I can safely say that the health benefits far outweigh the momentary cravings for food.

Not to mention, one of the great things about fasting is that it can and should be tailored to your specific needs and health concerns.

Why fast?

- Your body was specifically designed for periods of feast and famine
- Helps to normalize insulin levels—in turn utilizing more fat as fuel
- Normalizes hunger hormone
- Lowers triglyceride levels
- Decreases free radicals in the blood stream
- Longer lifespan
- Helps break food addiction patterns

- Detoxification
- Self-enlightenment and mental clarity
- Increased energy levels

So now that we've covered many of the benefits of fasting…what *type* of fast is right for you? Well, there are several different types of fasts— water, juice, brown rice. As a beginner, if it's warm outside I recommend starting with a juice fast. If it's winter then I recommend a brown rice fast. I would save water fasts for either one- or two-day periods if you're just starting out since they're much more difficult and taxing on the body.

The length of time will vary depending on your body's needs. To start out, simply commit to one full 24-hour period in which you only consumer juice or brown rice. If you're body is up to it and you feel mentally prepared, then feel free to keep going.

It's important to note, though that for the first 3 or so days you probably won't feel all that great. In fact, you'll most likely feel like death. Don't worry, though it's just all part of the detox symptoms which is one of the main reasons you should do a fast.

If you're finding it hard to continue on through those first few days you can attempt to alleviate some of the detox symptoms by soaking in an Epsom salt bath or performing an enema a couple times a day.

Keep in mind that just because you are fasting it doesn't mean you should use it as an excuse to avoid any activity whatsoever. Obviously, you probably shouldn't attempt to do anything at such a high-intensity level that you feel dizzy, but you should practice your daily asanas and meditate as well as go on long, relaxing walks.

Another helpful idea is to do a type of intermittent fasting (there are five different styles), called Eat Stop Eat which is a type of lifestyle diet in which you simply choose one day a week (doesn't matter which one) and abstain from eating for a full 24 hours.

By fasting one day a week, in a year's time you will have fasted for 52 days of the year. Pretty impressive results for not a lot of effort, considering.

Not to mention, the clarity and lightness you feel from fasting has incredible benefits on your yoga practice that you probably have never been able to experience before.

Try it for yourself. I promise you'll be glad you did!

Hack 3: Create a Morning Ritual

Creating a morning ritual might seem like an act that's reserved only for the most anally retentive types of people, but I promise it provides huge benefits for virtually everyone—especially yogis.

I don't know about you, but my day is a million times better when I start it off on the right foot. It seems like a no-brainer, right? Well, by developing a morning ritual and sticking to it, you're pretty much guaranteeing that your day will be positive and productive.

My personal morning ritual involves waking up just before sunrise to sip on some warm lemon water or hot ginger tea—focusing on the moment of quiet and stillness. After that, I do my rounds of sun salutations followed by meditation and affirmations.

Even if I don't accomplish anything else toward my yoga practice during the day, I take comfort and peace in the fact that I've done my sun salutations and meditation and don't feel quite so bad.

In fact, it tends to energize me and help me focus on the task that's at hand for the rest of the day. By developing a morning ritual I have ensured that I am much more accomplished and happy throughout my day and that alone is worth the sacrifice of waking up slightly earlier.

I'm not saying you have to wake up with the sunrise (although it's very rewarding), but I do encourage you to get in the habit of having a morning ritual or routine that you hold yourself accountable for.

The increase in productivity and happiness is well worth it!

Hack 4: Feng Shui Your Environment

Feng Shui might not be the first thing that comes to your mind when talking about yoga hacks, but it has its place and reasoning.

Traditionally speaking it's an ancient Chinese practice of laws that are designed to govern the spatial arrangement and orientation in a home in relation to the flow of energy (or qi).

However, there's also a similar practice in Hindu culture called Vastu Shastra—which roughly translates to 'home teachings.' Although both feng shui and vastu shastra originate in different parts of the world they are founded on similar beliefs: that there is a science to the prosperity and harmony in our homes and architectural structures and ways that we can enhance the positive energy and release the negative energy.

When talking about vastu shastra (and feng shui) if a dwelling or structure is not constructed with the rules and principles in mind to promote positive energy, then the people inside these structures will not be productive or harmonious. Simply by not having the foresight to arrange the structure or its contents in a positive and thoughtful way can have serious consequences, including: physical illness, loss of money and even untimely death.

Vastu shastra's origins come from ancient India, where people believed that houses were living organisms and as such, performed sacred ceremonies when constructing their homes.

Obviously, today many of us rent houses or live in apartments and don't have the ability to build a home from the ground up. However, there are ways to improve energy and functionality simply by arranging the contents inside your dwelling based on feng shui philosophy.

Here are some simple tips:

- Get rid of clutter
- Keep the toilet lid down
- Avoid working with your back to a door
- If it's broken—get rid of it
- Get some plants
- Keep a water source (i.e. fountain, mini pond, birdbath) near the entrance to your home—this attracts wealth
- Don't put your bed—or couch—directly in front of or facing away from a doorway

These might not seem like life changing tips, but the idea is to start small. And even if you don't believe in it at first, I encourage you to still give these things a try. After all, the objects and energy of our homes reflect our inner mind. What does yours say about you?

If you're not happy with the answer, the good news is it's never too late to make changes and create the energy you want your home to reflect.

Hack 5: Go on a Yoga Retreat

This one might seem obvious, but I find that most people tend to overlook this option and I'm not sure why. I know that when I was first starting out in my yoga practice I was a little intimidated at the thought of going to a yoga retreat.

Maybe because it brought to mind images of naked hippies doing crazy hard pretzel poses while I looked on and felt left out—obviously back then I wasn't too enlightened.

Eventually, though, I got my courage up and went to my first yoga retreat in college. It was a weekend retreat and it ended up being one of the most memorable and unforgettable yoga experiences I've ever had. I even ended up making some incredible like-minded friends that I am still close to, to this day.

If you're worried about taking the plunge—I urge you to get over that fear. Whatever image you've built up in your mind, I promise it's nothing like that. If you just don't feel comfortable jumping head first into a situation where you don't know anyone (like me), then make a friend or two come along with you.

I'd just like to say, though that some of the best experiences come from when we let ourselves be the most vulnerable. So if you can go it alone, I suggest doing so. You'll meet so many new people and have a ton of fun. It can be a day, a weekend or even a week or two—just get out of your comfort zone and expand your mind.

Hack 6: Expect Nothing

This is truly one of the hardest parts of yoga to master. Logically and fundamentally speaking—it makes sense. But yet, when our bodies are incapable of doing a pose in the manner in which we think it should be able to…that's a whole 'nother story, isn't it?

I remember quite a few years ago I was hit by a car while crossing at a crosswalk. Although I was lucky I didn't break any bones, the accident put me (and my yoga practice) out of commission for several months.

As I slowly eased back into things through Pilates-based physical therapy I remember being so disappointed that I no longer felt as flexible as I had been prior to all of this happening. I couldn't do Forward Bend without a sharp searing pain in my lower back and I sure as heck couldn't touch my forehead to my shins like I had been able to do previously.

I'd like to say I handled the situation with grace, but it really derailed me for awhile and I felt like all my hard work had been for nothing.

The beauty of the situation was, though, that it forced me to really fight for what I wanted and to re-assess my beliefs about my body and my life. After a few months had passed I picked myself up, brushed myself off and got back on the saddle. Of course, I was starting over from square one basically at that point, but it felt good.

I was able to really focus on the moment and let me expectations be pushed aside to make way for whatever positive energy and life change was coming my way.

Now, I'm not saying that I want you to go get yourself into some horrible accident to improve your mindfulness capabilities. But I do want to remind you that there are many things in our lives that are out of our control.

Yes, our bodies are one of those things. We might feel like we can make it do whatever we want, but usually when we try to force ourselves into stretches and poses we aren't ready for it ends up backfiring and we're out of commission for a few days.

You just never know when there may come a day when you're no longer capable of doing a certain stretch that you've been beating yourself up over—and you'd give anything to get back to where you used to be.

So basically, all this is to say that I encourage you to start each session of your yoga practice with positive intention and respect for your body's capabilities and limits—and love it because of and in spite of them.

Hack 7: Take it Outside

Your yoga practice, that is. If you haven't given outdoor yoga a proper chance, the time is now! There are so many amazing benefits to it that it's kind of insane.

Why should you practice yoga outside?

- Helps you to connect with nature and Mother Earth
- Makes your breathing more productive
- Lets you deepen your postures
- Gives you a boost of Vitamin D
- Promotes better self-awareness
- Increases happiness
- Offers a challenge to poses you're comfortable with

If you do decide to give outdoor yoga a try (which I encourage you to!) then here are a few tips for you.

A few things to keep in mind:

- You may want to get a mat just for use outside
- Pick a good spot—away from hot sun, poison ivy, tree roots and lots of distractions

- Be sure to slather on the SPF and use bug deterrent (preferably not bug spray)
- If you're going to do yoga at the beach—do your poses closer to the water since the sand will be more compact and less likely to cause injury
- Practice being mindful of nature while you're going through your poses
- Try a class—if you're intimidated of doing solo yoga in a public place for fear of looking like a crazy person, test the waters in a group session

Once you get comfortable practicing outdoors, don't be surprised if doing yoga in a studio setting is no longer as appealing.

Connecting to nature on such a deep level as you do through yoga practice is very therapeutic and addicting. What are you waiting for? Give it a try for yourself.

Hack 8: Discover Your Dosha(s)

There are three Ayurvedic Doshas (or, mind-body types): they are Vata, Pitta and Kapha. The majority of us will have a predominant dosha, while a select few will have two dominant doshas.

Doshas are simply types of energy that circulate throughout the body and control our physiological activity. They are made up of five elements: space, air, fire, water and earth and each of these elements combine in different ways to form our three constitutional principles— or doshas.

Basically, they're responsible for the traits of our body, mind and spirit.

The **Vata dosha** is comprised of space and air and controls our movement.

The **Pitta dosha** is comprised of fire and water and controls metabolism and digestion.

The **Kapha dosha** is comprised of water and earth and controls our structure and stability.

At different points in our lives our dominant dosha(s) will fluctuate and change and we'll have varying degrees of all three at any given moment. However, it's important for us to try and target our dominant dosha in relation to our yoga practice and dietary choices. The reason being is because this helps keep our energy balanced and our body functioning at its optimal level.

The first step in this process is to find out which of your doshas is the most dominant and then to get everything back into balance. The best way to do that is by taking a quiz to help you figure it out.

There are plenty around the internet if you Google 'dosha quiz' but my favorite one can be found at **http://doshaquiz.chopra.com**

It was developed by Deepak Chopra and is really in-depth. It has multiple parts to help you figure out your dominant dosha and also to determine where you're imbalanced and offers advice on how to solve this dilemma.

Once you've determined your dominant dosha you'll be able to cater your eating habits and yoga practice to fit your own personal mind-body type needs.

Hack 9: Lay on a Bed of Nails

No, I don't mean a literal bed of nails (although it's not nearly as scary as you think it would be). I'm actually talking about a new product invented for yoga and meditation purposes.

And did you know that the original idea of a bed of nails originated in Asia over 1,000 years ago? It is also believed to have been used by the gurus and yogis of ancient India for healing and meditation purposes.

But if I'm not referring to an actual bed of nails, then what the heck do I mean? Well, there's a relatively new, life-changing product on the market that is specifically targeted towards yogis. It's a mat (that you can also get with a matching pillow if you like) that provides benefits in the comfort of your own home that are similar to acupuncture.

The mat is designed with small, non-toxic plastic discs all over it with multiple little "spikes" on each disc. The pressure it produces against your skin actually helps to release endorphins, oxytocin and even energy and pain relief.

This is really exciting, because even though it doesn't necessarily replace the act of getting acupuncture performed, it's a much more affordable at-home option that you can use regularly to supplement some of the benefits you'd be paying hundreds for, otherwise.

According to the Bed of Nails website: http://bodofnails.org their product (with regular and prolonged use) helps:

- Reduce blood pressure
- Improve skin
- Reduce anxiety and stress
- Benefit weight loss
- Relieve constipation
- Improve circulation
- Get rid of headaches
- Relieve chronic pain in the neck and back
- Improve sleep and insomnia

I personally own one (as do several of my friends) and I honestly couldn't live without the thing now. It really has helped me to be more relaxed and it does improve my overall sense of happiness and calm after I use it—and no, I'm not getting paid to say that.

If you're looking for a way to make your meditation or savasana more beneficial give Bed of Nails a try.

Hack 10: Do Aerial Yoga at Home

This is one of my favorite at-home yoga discoveries ever! If you're even remotely interested in acro-yoga, aerial yoga or just have a sense of adventure and like hanging around…then you absolutely *have* to try out a yoga swing for yourself.

The only brand of yoga swing that I use and recommend is the Omni Gym. These were the swings I was first introduced to when I was taking aerial yoga classes in New York while in college and it was love at first swing.

The good thing about the Omni Gym brand is that they have lots (and lots) of different models to fit every type of budget. I mean, obviously the Omni Gym Complete is top-notch, but if that's out of your price range then there are more affordable and more compact options.

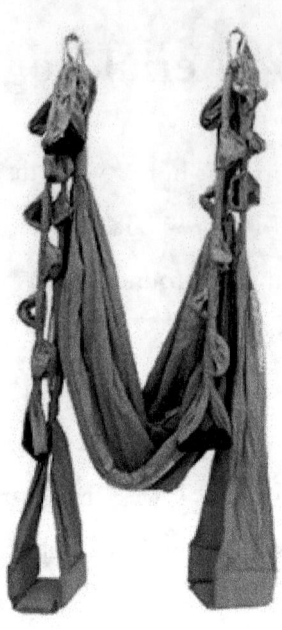

The Omni Swing Basic

(in Lavender)

I actually own the Omni Gym Complete that I use in my at-home studio and then I also own a few Omni Swing Basics—one in my bedroom and one in my living room. The good thing about these swings is that they come in lots of different, fun colors so you can match it to your décor if you want. Plus, I find that they make for great conversation because when I have people over they're always curious about what the contraption is hanging from my living room ceiling.

And yes, they always want to try it out and end up loving it.

I'm not being paid by Omni Gym to say these things about their products—I just really love all their products and couldn't imagine my life without them. Like I said, they have lots of options that fit every budget and you really can't beat the convenience of being able to practice aerial yoga from the comfort of your own home.

Be sure to check them out if you're interested.

Hack 11: Foam Roll!

Remember the accident I told you about, where I got hit by a car? Well, as a result of that accident and having to go to physical therapy I actually discovered the amazing benefits of foam rolling.

If you're not familiar with the topic of foam rolling I'll break it down for you: it's simply self-massage (think deep tissue) using a cylindrical piece of solid foam.

What Are the Benefits?

- Helps lengthen tight muscles, ligaments and tendons
- Improves circulation for better cellular function (i.e. aids in detox)
- Promotes better range of motion in the spine
- Improves blood flow to the skin and muscles that you're working on
- Increases flexibility

Picking out a foam roller can be kind of overwhelming; there are so many choices. Not to mention they come in different lengths and shapes. Generally though, the longer the better—as you can work out the tension in larger areas of your body with it. The one that I own is, I believe 36" in length and that's the longest one I've ever seen.

When you're picking out a foam roller you also want to look for one that's advertised as 'high density.' This basically just means that it can handle more weight per cubic foot—which means it won't have much give and you'll get a better quality "massage" out of it. Not to mention it should last for a long time.

Also, just as a note: you're going to see lots of different designs of foam rollers with geometric Tetris-like patterned bumps sticking up on the surfaces. Although it might look exciting and like a good idea to purchase a foam roller with lots of bumps on the surface I don't really recommend it. Especially if you have tight muscles or are just beginning with foam rolling. It causes a lot of unnecessary pain without much added benefit. I promise that just a standard cylindrical foam roller works wonders and provides amazing benefits—and you'll actually be more likely to want to keep using it since it isn't quite as pain-inducing.

By using a foam roller regularly (I recommend doing it nightly before bed) you will improve your range of motion in your asanas and also be more flexible in every day activities.

Hack 12: Balance Your Chakras

So before you can balance your chakras, maybe you need to know what they even are. Below you'll find a diagram that details all seven chakras in your body.

Basically, each chakra is just a spinning "wheel" of energy that is responsible for certain traits and dictating our prana—or life force. Our chakras are what keep us healthy, vibrant and *alive*.

Whether you're aware of it or not, each of your chakras are hard at work every day to keep your body, mind and spirit running smoothly. However, sometimes energy deficiencies cause one or all of our chakras to become "blocked" and not operate at their optimal levels.

When chakras become out of balance a number of problems can occur depending on which chakra(s) is out of whack. Below you can see where each chakra is located in relation to your body.

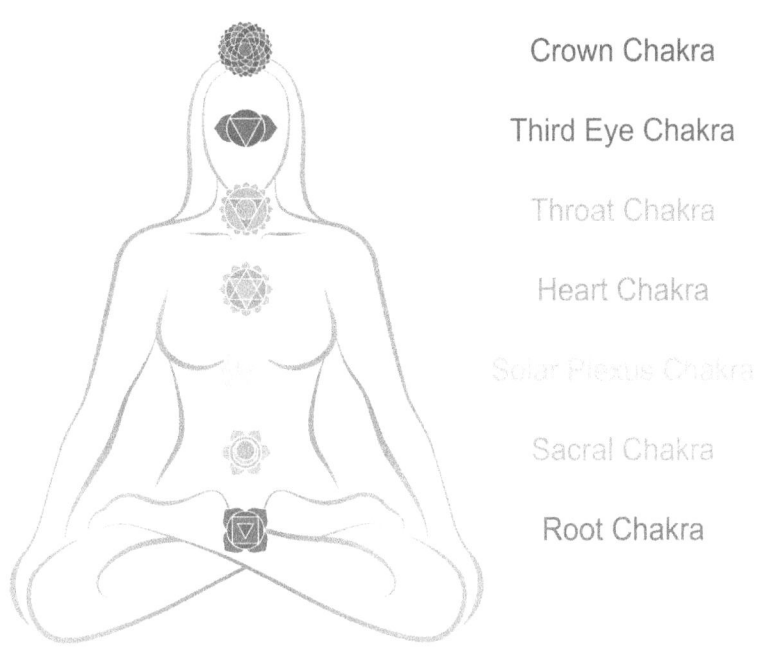

Crown Chakra

Third Eye Chakra

Throat Chakra

Heart Chakra

Solar Plexus Chakra

Sacral Chakra

Root Chakra

The first Chakra is your Root Chakra, then on up the length of the spine to Chakra #7—the Crown Chakra.

I won't go into all the details of each specific chakra and what they're in charge of—I'd have to write a whole 'nother book. However, if you're interested in more details you can check out my book Yoga With a Purpose that goes over each specific chakra and how they function within our bodies.

As for right now, though, for simplicity's sake we'll just go over how to balance them once they're off kilter.

1) **Root Chakra**—The best type of healing you can do for your first and "base" chakra is participating in physical activities—think yoga. The reason being is because this chakra is most related to our physical body. You can also get lots of benefit from aromatherapy treatments because the base chakra relates well to our sense of smell as well as gemstones since this chakra is the earth element.

2) **Sacral Chakra**—The second chakra is our sexual center and is also a very physical part of our bodies. You can use tantric yoga (especially) to tap into your sacral chakra and unleash your intimacy. You can also try healing this chakra with specific foods since it's related to your sense of taste.

3) **Solar Plexus Chakra**—Our solar plexus chakra is incredibly visual, so things like affirmations and yantras are especially beneficial to tapping into this chakra. Not to mention, sun bathing or fire walking since the third chakra is connected to the element of fire.

4) **Heart Chakra**—The fourth chakra is considered the bridge between our upper and lower chakras—it connects our physical selves to our spiritual selves. Because of this, touch is an amazing heart chakra opener. Simply practicing self-hugging has tremendous healing benefits for the fourth chakra. You can also practice tapping or EFT as well as breath work since the heart chakra's element is air.

5) **Throat Chakra**—To tap into and unblock your fifth chakra, the best way to go is through sound therapy—either hearing sounds or

performing sounds. This means you can chant, sing or say mantras or simply take sounds in through mantras, your favorite song or even crystal bowls or gongs.

6) **Third Eye Chakra**—Since our sixth chakra is considered our third eye, visualization is the prime way to tap into it and unblock it. Practice visualizing your goals and dreams each day and focus specifically on *feeling* these visions as if they've already happened.

7) **Crown Chakra**—The last chakra is incredibly spiritual and is focused on the practice of meditation. Think silent, thoughtless forms of meditation in savasana. Focus only on opening your mind and body up to the openness of the space you're in—nothing else.

I encourage you to try lots of different techniques and ideas for opening up each specific chakra. Just because a specific practice helps open up your friend's third chakra doesn't mean it will have the same affect on yours. Just like anything else in our bodies our chakras are highly individual to us and respond to different things. So have fun and experiment to find what works best for you.

Please note that when a chakra is off balance you're going to want to avoid doing what is going to be best for healing that specific chakra. So just because you don't necessarily *want* to do something doesn't mean you *shouldn't.*

Hack 13: Remember to Smile

This might seem like an incredibly simple hack, but it's highly beneficial to your yoga practice.

Think about it: smiling is generally something you do when you feel relaxed, happy, light, at ease. Right? This is exactly the same way you should feel when you're practicing yoga. So theoretically you should be smiling throughout your entire session.

However, that's not usually the case. So many times I look up in class only to find students so focused and stressed out that they're hardly even breathing, let alone smiling. Generally, the first thing to go when you're starting to feel the pressure is your smile.

This isn't necessarily a bad thing, though: it's an easy way for us to gauge where we're at mentally while we're practicing our asanas. If you find that you're frowning or furrowing your brow in frustration in your pose then gently check in and remind yourself to relax and have some fun—don't take it too seriously.

Hack 14: Lemons and Your Mat

Is your yoga mat getting a little dingy and you're not sure how to clean it? Should you just go buy a new one? Definitely not. I'm pretty sure this hack will basically change your life. But why lemons? Well, they're great all-natural cleaners for nearly any surface because they're antibacterial and acidic. Plus, as an added bonus they smell great!

I came up with this little trick when I was living in my tiny apartment in New York. So if you're like me, or other city yogis who have very little space to work with (or simply just want an easier way to clean your mat) then you'll love this trick. I personally use a variation of this to clean the studio mats and it does a great job.

What You'll Need:

1 Lemon

A dirty yoga mat

Scrubby sponge

Organic soap

Water

Lint-free towel

First, grab your lemon and cut it in half (lengthwise). On one side of your mat, squeeze one half of the lemon all over the surface.

Next, grab your scrubby sponge and put a few drops of soap on it and get it wet. Rub the sponge all over the surface of your mat with the lemon juice on it.

Then, simply rinse the sponge off and clear the soap off the surface of your mat.

Repeat the same process on the opposite side of your mat and then towel dry both sides to help it dry even faster.

Hack 15: Set a Dedicated Time to Practice

This hack is pretty simple and straightforward, but if you put it into effect it can have a huge impact on the quality of your yoga practice.

Think about it: if you're constantly having to stress over when and *if* you're going to get your practice in for the day, needless to say it can make the whole yoga experience less than zen.

So what if by simply changing one small habit you were able to simplify and de-stress your entire yoga experience? Would you do it? I would like to think so.

How about for just **one week** you set a specific time of day (right when you wake up, for example) to do your yoga practice. Make sure you also define how long you're going to do it each day—preferably at least 30 minutes or more—and stick to it.

No matter what happens, don't let yourself stray from your new routine. After a week you'll be able to see the major benefits of having a set time for your yoga practice guaranteed.

Once you've tried doing it this way I highly doubt you'll want to go back to the stress of the *when* and *if* yoga routine.

Hack 16: Get Grounded

The premise of grounding or "earthing" is that by walking barefoot on the surface of the earth and being in direct contact with grass, soil, sand or water you're receiving "electrical nutrition" straight from the magnetic field of the earth.

Whether you necessary believe this to be true or not, you can't deny the amazing feeling or "charge" you get by being barefoot at the beach or walking barefoot in plush green grass. This is grounding—a subtle and natural energy we get directly from the earth that helps us to "recharge" our body's circuitry and biological rhythms.

Obviously, this has major benefits and powerful healing effects that help improve sleep, reduce pain and inflammation and create a feeling of calmness.

But the problem is, with our modern lifestyles we are becoming increasingly disconnected from the earth. Think about it: in historic times we used to walk around barefoot much more often (in prehistoric times, always) and sleep on the ground, which helped us to re-connect with the earth daily.

Now, it's rare if we ever do those things.

If you want to improve your health and overall feeling of well-being then there are some simple things you can do to practice "earthing."

Modern Earthing

- Do yoga barefoot in the grass or on the sand
- Go for a walk on the beach (barefoot, obviously)
- Take your shoes and socks off when you go to the park and walk or sit in the grass for awhile—especially if it's dew-y
- Get an earthing mat to sleep on—it helps to conduct electrons from the earth to your body
- Go swimming in the ocean or a lake
- Purchase grounding shoes—my personal favorites are Juil's brand

Now that you know the why and the how, you don't have any excuse—go get grounded! The health benefits don't have to be seen or understood, even, to be *felt*.

Hack 17: Read the *Yoga Sutras*

Most likely, you love everything about yoga—you live it, breathe it, practice it, but yet...you haven't read the foundational texts of the origins of yoga.

Believe me, I get that it probably isn't that enticing to read Patanjali's *Yoga Sutras*. After all, it was written nearly 5,000 years ago and in Sanskrit nonetheless.

Did you know, though, that there is a fairly modern translation that was written by Swami Satchidananda? It was first published in 1978, but has since been revised and updated numerous times.

Even if history isn't your thing, if you want to take your yoga practice to a new level, I think it's imperative to know *where* yoga comes from—and this is the most accessible way to do that.

I encourage you to give it a read. Who knows, it might help you create a deeper mind-body connection and will only better your understanding of how modern yoga came to be.

Hack 18: Say No to Cotton and Hot Yoga

If you've ever attended a Bikram yoga class, then you know it gets...*hot*. Okay, to be more precise, roughly 104 degrees Fahrenheit with a humidity of 40%...for 90 minutes.

Yeah! So your clothing of choice when going to a hot yoga class is vitally important. Most people prefer to wear as skimpy of clothes as possible since you're going to be basically swimming in your own sweat (and maybe other peoples', too).

Just a little helpful hint: never wear anything cotton! At all. It becomes incredibly heavy and drenched in sweat and makes it very hard to move into your postures easily. It's just added weight and an extra obstacle you don't need.

The best clothing of choice for Bikram is moisture-wicking and form-fitting types of clothing. Think polyester microfiber blends, spandex and lycra.

Generally, most workout clothes are made from these materials, but check the label before you get your sweat on, just to be sure.

Hack 19: Yoga Classes on the Cheap

Most of us can use a little help when it comes to money and even if we aren't dirt poor, we like the idea of saving a little cash when we can.

Plus, it's no secret that individual yoga classes can be quite price-y. One of the best ways to get around this if you don't have a lot of money to dedicate to your practice, is by find free or discounted classes in your area.

Most yoga studios will offer a free or highly discounted "pass" to new, potential members that are generally good for about a week's worth of classes. Most of the time these can be used on any number of classes and are unlimited so you can try out as many classes as you want.

This is especially beneficial for those who aren't sure what type of yoga will best suit their needs and personal yogic style. You can also get insanely good deals at most studios if you're a student. Lucky you!

If you happen to live near a Lululemon store they actually offer "the gift of yoga" (free classes) weekly at their stores. Check with your local store for times and dates.

Along the same lines, if you live in a bigger city, chances are there are community yoga classes being taught somewhere. These can be outdoors or at community centers and they're usually advertised on Craigslist, the newspaper or local community websites. They're usually free, donation-based, or super-cheap.

If you currently have a gym membership, check to see if your gym offers complimentary fitness classes. Chances are if they do they have some sort of yoga class you can take as part of your membership. Although these don't tend to be as zen-focused they're a good option if you're on a budget.

Another idea is to organize your own yoga class, either with friends or coworkers. It doesn't have to be fancy, but it can be a great way for you to have the sense of community you get from taking a class at a studio—especially if you find like-minded people who share the same goals as you.

Hack 20: Improve the Quality of Your Sleep

If you're like the majority of the population your sleep quality could use some improving.

Now, if you're a yogi you're already a step ahead of the rest of the population because, as we all know, regular yoga practice improves our sleep habits and ability to be able to get a better night's sleep.

While that's true, there is usually still some room for improvement.

One of the big ways we **all** can improve upon our ability to get to sleep easily and actually *stay* asleep throughout the night is to cut back on our after dark use of technology. The reason being is because the screens on our iPads, computers, smart phones and other devices emit large amounts of blue light that actually alters how sleepy we feel and how alert we are and even suppresses our melatonin levels. Not to mention, the quality of our REM sleep is much worse when we are reading or working on a computer screen before bed.

Obviously the most ideal situation would be to cut out the technology use several hours before bed to ensure proper sleeping patterns.

However, I get that that's not possible for everyone—including me.

So there are a few hacks you can use to counteract the negative drawbacks of using technology in regards to your sleep.

The first tip is to wear a pair of blue-light blocking "safety" glasses if you're going to be working on a computer or reading or looking at another device a few hours before bed. The glasses you would need to wear are actually orange and cancel out the blue lights that disrupt our sleep.

You can find a suitable pair here on Amazon, but you should also be able to find them in any home improvement store as well.

If you personally find the idea of wearing bright orange safety glasses unappealing, I totally get it and I've got you covered.

One of the best alternative solutions I've found is a free software called f.lux. The premise is that you simply download it onto your computer (it's compatible for both Mac OS and Windows), tell it what your time zone is and when you wake up and f.lux takes care of the rest.

Basically, the software adjusts your computer screen's brightness throughout the day so that no matter what time you're working you are reducing the amount of blue light you're exposing your eyes to. During the day it looks fairly normal, but as the evening goes on and especially after dark you'll see a noticeable orange tint to your screen.

It's simple and effective and I highly recommend giving it a try. After using the software for a week you should notice a huge difference in your sleep. Oh, and if you're not sure if you're able to tell a difference in the brightness—switch it off for a few at night to see the dramatic change in color.

You can download f.lux for free at https://justgetflux.com

Hack 21: Take Your Own Yoga Pictures

We're all familiar with the act of taking a selfie (even though I hate that word!). Thanks to modern technology we are able to share our faces with the rest of the world through Facebook and Instagram and other social networking sites.

The same goes for yogis who like to take pictures of themselves. But…what do you do when your hands are all tied up and you can't hold your phone? How are you supposed to be able to concentrate on the positioning of your Peacock pose when you're having to worry about how to take your own picture?

Well the obvious answer is that you could just have someone else take the picture for you. But we all know that sometimes you just want to take 100 and pick the best one. And most friends or family members don't want to be your personal photographer all hours of the day.

The solution? Helpful smart phone apps that have timer settings and capabilities so you don't have to stand there with your finger on the button each time or ask someone else to do it for you.

Some of my favorite apps are Camera Timer and VSCO Cam (which is an editing app).

Camera Timer is…you guessed it: a timer app that lets you set it to various time lengths before it takes the shots. However, one of my favorite things about it is that you can choose a multiple photo option so that it takes a number of consecutive shots of your choosing so you're much more likely to get a better picture of yourself. This app also lets you select a 'period'—or length of time between each photo that's taken, which is also a plus.

Another (safer) option is to take a video of your yoga session and either take stills from the video or post part of the video itself.

If you're going to go the app and self-timer route, I suggest purchasing a tripod or using a phone stand to keep your phone in position. Otherwise you're either most likely going to end up with a cracked screen or spend many precious minutes out of your practice to keep sitting it back upright because it fell.

Remember: the goal of your yoga practice is peace and inner calm. If whatever you're doing isn't helping with that then it probably isn't a worthwhile endeavor.

Hack 22: Get the Right Accessories

This one is pretty simple, but for some reason a lot of people overlook it—especially if they've been practicing for quite awhile.

Many times when we're experienced we tend to let our egos get in the way of utilizing things that could help enhance or make our practice easier. In a way we view it as cheating, I think. I'm here to say, though, there are days (even after 13+ years) that I still use a block or two or a bolster. There ain't no shame in my game!

We really need to start listening to our bodies more and our ego less. A way to do this is by using the right accessories that will help enhance our practice in a positive way and keep us moving forward.

Here are some of my favorite products:

- Blocks
- Yoga socks
- Yoga gloves
- Bolsters
- Foam roller
- Yoga towel (to go over your mat—especially great for Hot Yoga)

Some of these things might seem unnecessary to those with some experience in their yoga practice. But I can assure you that there's never anything to be ashamed of if you feel like you could use a little extra help in some areas.

Hack 23: Subscribe to an Online Yoga Class

Practicing yoga at home is one of my favorite ways to do it. It's peaceful, relaxing and everything yoga should be. If you like to practice at home, but are running out of impromptu yoga routines or just aren't feeling inspired—try taking a yoga class online.

There are plenty of free sources for yoga routines and even more paid resources.

Here are some of my favorite free sites:

- www.yogabycandace.com
- www.yogawithadriene.com
- www.doyogawithme.com
- www.myfreeyoga.com
- www.myyogaworks.com

Here are some of my favorite paid sites:

- www.gaiamtv.com
- www.yogaglo.com

- www.yogavibes.com
- www.yogatoday.com

Obviously this is not an exhaustive list. The internet is a vast and wide place with lots of possibilities—these are just some of my personal favorites.

If you don't find what you're looking for here try checking YouTube. You'd be surprised what you can get for free on there.

Hack 24: Master the Mudras

Just like we talked about before when we discussed connecting with our dominant dosha type, our physical body is made up of those five elements: water, air, fire, earth and space.

When any of these elements are imbalanced our entire body system is compromised and disrupted.

Mudras—or, symbolic hand gestures—can be used to reconnect one part of our body to another and restore balance within our bodies. It is believed that by utilizing mudras you ignite an electromagnetic current inside your body that helps to cure imbalances.

Each of our fingers has a respectful element tied to it. They are as follows.

1) Thumb = fire
2) Index = air
3) Middle = space
4) Ring = earth
5) Pinky = water

There are many many different mudras that can be and are used in the practice of yoga to connect our mind and body and help restore prana (or life force) back into our bodies.

If you want to delve deeper into your yoga practice I highly suggest using mudras to help balance all aspects of your life.

Hack 25: Cheap and Stylish Yoga Clothes

I hate to admit it, but one of my more dominant passions in life is finding cute, but affordable yoga clothes. It excites me. I think that everyone who practices yoga deserves to feel *and* look good in the clothes that they wear.

Everyone *knows* and *loves* Lululemon—and for good reason: their pieces are stylish and well-made and are super comfortable. The problem is, though, I hate spending $100 on a single pair of yoga pants. I mean, is that really necessary?

So in this hack I'm going to provide you with a list of fun places that offer cute yoga clothes to the masses at great prices.

Here are some maybe not-so-obvious places to look:

- Forever21
- Old Navy
- Fabletics
- Target

- Gap
- Nordstrom Rack
- TJ Maxx (sold only in stores)
- Marshall's (sold only in stores)

My personal favorites are Forever21 and Fabletics. With Forever21 they offer incredibly cute clothes at super-cheap prices. Fabletics, though, offers awesome quality for mid-range prices and even offers a new outfit a month for a good deal.

So no, you don't have to spend upwards of $200 to get a completely cute yoga outfit to feel good in. You're welcome!

Hack 26: 30 Day Challenge

This is simple enough in terms of what it is—however implementing it can be an entirely different beast.

I challenge you to take a 30 day hiatus from technology and see what it does for your yoga practice.

Yes, you heard me. Spend 30 whole days without using your computer, smart phone (other than for talking on the phone), tablet, TV or any other distracting device.

During these 30 days you're welcome to read actual books, write on actual paper and use your phone for its intended purpose (talking, not texting). You'll have to get creative and it will also force you to become more centered to your mind-body connection.

I promise if you commit to this for 30 days, after a week you'll start seeing huge changes in the depth of your yoga practice and how clear your mind becomes.

Now, I understand that for some people it's literally impossible to perform this challenge at 100% due to being a student or job constraints. So if you can't do the full monty then at least cut out all social media outlets (think Instagram, Facebook, Tinder etc.).

It's definitely not going to be easy and you'll probably hate me for a good two weeks, but at the end you'll feel a huge sense of accomplishment and pride for what you've done.

Hack 27: Practice Pranayama

If you've been practicing yoga for any length of time at all then I'm sure you know what pranayama is. But how often do you actually focus on it and do it correctly?

In case you have no idea what I'm talking about, pranayama is simply the practice of certain breathing exercises and techniques—especially as they relate to different asanas.

I'm sure you know that breathing is an integral part to practicing yoga effectively, but you might not know exactly *why* that's the case.

Well, this is where pranayama comes in: it's actually the fourth limb of Patanjali's Eight Limbs of Yoga and it's basically a way for us to control our vital life force—or prana while at the same time cleansing our mind and body.

Generally speaking there are many many different types of yogic breathing exercises depending on which form of yoga you're practicing. However, in Western culture there are a few main ones that are more predominant during yoga classes.

Popular Pranayama Techniques

1) Alternate Nostril Breathing
2) Light Skull Breathing
3) Ocean Breath
4) Three-Part Breath
5) Breath of Fire

Generally speaking, these practices are best learned through the guidance of a trained teacher or professional, but you can also teach yourself if you find proper videos online from a trusted source.

Hack 28: Create a Sacred Yoga Space at Home

If you don't have an at-home yoga practice then now is the time to start one. And if you do, then now is the time to tailor it and make it into a sacred and special space in your home that is dedicated to your yoga practice and goals.

Practicing yoga at home is one of the most rewarding ways to get more out of each yoga session—especially after you've mastered all the basics. I just find it to be much more zen and peaceful, but maybe that's because I'm just introverted.

Either way, if you consider yourself a serious yogi and want to take it to the next level then I highly recommend that you dedicate a specific part of your home, only to your yoga practice.

Fill it with items that are meaningful to you and create a calm, cozy and relaxed environment where you can connect and grow with your higher Self.

Some things you might include:

- Candles

- Comfortable pillows

- Soft or natural lighting

- Essential oil diffuser

- Positive affirmations

- Tranquil and calming music

- Art that inspires you

Whatever you decide to include should make it a place where you feel 100% comfortable and open, away from the distractions of everyday life. By taking the time to carve out a special place solely for your yoga practice you're taking it one step further on your path to mind-body connection.

Hack 29: Try Something New

When it comes to yoga there are so many different types that it can be overwhelming and very easy to fall into a pattern of only practicing a specific type that you've come to know and love.

While I think that it's amazing to get so connected to a practice that you truly love, I also think it's important to keep growing and changing to ensure that your energy stays balanced.

Ideas for changing it up:

- Aerial yoga
- Kundalini yoga
- SUP yoga (Stand Up Paddleboard—it's done *on* the water)
- Outdoor yoga
- Transcendental Meditation
- Hot yoga
- Tantra yoga
- Yin yoga

So the next time you get a chance to try a different type of yoga that you wouldn't normally consider, give it a second thought. You never know: it might be just what you your mind and body need.

Hack #30: Develop Your Own Special Mantra

The way we think and feel about ourselves day in and day out has a very profound impact on our success in life.

There's an old saying that states, "Mantras are energy which can be likened to fire. Fire can cook your lunch or burn down the forest."

And it's incredibly true: if you constantly think the worst then most likely you're going to get it. But how can we change this? If we are just naturally pessimistic and negative isn't that that? Nope.

Traditionally speaking, in Hindu and Buddhist cultures a mantra is defined as a sound or word repeated to help aid in concentration while meditating. Today, however we use mantras for many different purposes—not just while meditating.

Mantras, similar to affirmations, are incredibly important phrases or words that we can use in our daily lives to change the way we feel, become empowered and even bring dreams to fruition.

What are some examples of mantras?

- OM—one of the more popular yoga mantras.
- I open my body and my heart to others and the Universe.
- Let (your name) be (your name)—for example: Let Olivia be Olivia.
- I am kindhearted and want the best for myself and others.
- I am doing the best that I can.

So now that you have a little inspiration, it's time to create a personal mantra just for you. Find someplace quiet, preferably out in nature on a sunny day. Take a pen and paper and begin by writing down all the positive thoughts that come to you. There's no need to think or filter these ideas out—simply write.

Now take all those words and ideas and thoughts that were given to you from your soul and compile them into one strong, powerful statement to empower you each day.

Say these words over and over again each day both in your mind and out loud to help feed your soul.

Hack #31: Incorporate the Yamas and Niyamas

Patanjali's Eight Limbs of Yoga included the Yamas and Niyamas—spiritual teachings and advice on how to treat yourself and the world around you.

Before we go any further with this, I'll quickly go over what they are.

The 5 Yamas

1) Ahimsa—non-violence.
2) Satya—truthfulness.
3) Asteya—non-stealing.
4) Brahmacharya—continence.
5) Aparigraha—non-covetousness.

The 5 Niyamas

1) Saucha—purification.
2) Santosha—contentment.
3) Tapas—asceticism.
4) Svadhyaya—self-study.
5) Ishvara Pranidhana—devotion.

So as you can see, his guidelines for how we live our lives are still quite relevant to us today. There's a reason he included the vows that he did for us to follow. Each one is specifically designed to improve our practice and overall way of living through our actions, thoughts and words.

By taking Patanjali's Yamas and Niyamas (and all the other Eight Limbs of Yoga) to heart you'll be able to open up your mind, body and spirit to a deeper connection with humanity and the Universe.

If you want more in-depth information on how to practice these guidelines in your everyday life (because there's a lot more to it) you can pick up my book Yoga With a Purpose to help you out on your spiritual yoga journey.

Hack #32: Adopt the Yogic Diet

Maybe you've been doing everything with your practice right, but when it comes to food you just can't seem to get yourself under control.

If you're finding it hard to change your eating habits or simply just want to get closer to yoga's traditional roots then you can start eating a sattvic diet—also known as the Yogic Diet.

In yoga tradition it's believed that the food we eat feeds our soul. What we consume (both for our mind and body) creates our prana to sustain our health and vitality.

The foundation to the sattvic diet is ahimsa (one of the 5 yamas), which teaches to practice non-harm to all other living things. Therefore, the sattvic diet denies eating foods that involve the killing or harming of animals.

By eating a yogic diet, we increase our prana and state of consciousness. The beauty of it is that anyone wanting to attain a higher spiritual path or healthier journey can easily follow it.

Approved Foods

- Fruit

- Vegetables—but no onions or garlic

- Legumes

- Whole grains

- Natural sugars (think maple syrup, molasses)

- Nuts and seeds

- Plant-based oil

- Spices that are sweet

- Herbal teas

- Food that is prepared with love

By following a sattvic diet—even if it isn't every single day of the week, you are contributing to a healthier life for yourself and the rest of the planet.

This is by no means, an exhaustive account of what the sattvic diet is, but it should get you well on your way to feeding your soul and your practice—one bite at a time.

Hack #33: Visit the Birthplace of Yoga

If you truly want to experience and discover yoga for what it really is, then you must, at some point in your life, visit India. After all, it *is* the birthplace of yoga.

Practicing yoga *in* India is about as close as you can get to sitting down and having a chat with Patanjali.

But be warned: it's not like it is here in Western culture—and for good reason. It has kept close to its traditional roots and continues to be more of a spiritual medium for practitioners, rather than an exercise regimen.

If you can, it's best to experience the Indian culture and yogic heritage through a specific yoga retreat. That way you aren't grappling around trying to figure out how to maneuver a new country while practicing yoga at the same time.

Retreats are a great way to experience new forms of yoga—especially when you're putting yourself directly in the middle of a culture that you probably aren't that familiar with.

Yoga is only part of India's story, but it is a great place to start and there's no better way to take your yoga practice to the next level, than to visit its birthplace.

Conclusion

So there you have it!

33 simple, yet life altering hacks to enhance your yoga practice.

At this point you may be feeling a bit overwhelmed at the information overload, which is understandable. Just try to remember that the goal here—as with most things in yoga—is to take it slow.

There is no rush to implement all or even *any* of these if you don't feel inclined to do so. But I think that you feel deep down that your yoga practice has more to give and so you sought out this book to help you with that.

I hope that the tips and techniques offered to you in this book have inspired you to take your yoga journey and turn it upside down—maybe even literally.

Remember: there's no right or wrong way to practice yoga. Follow your heart and let it be your guide to awakening your own true path to enlightenment and fulfillment through your practice.

Thanks for reading!